400∞

Haircutting
the Professional Way

Bruno

HAIRCUTTING

the Professional Way

Illustrations by Dany Simon
Translated by Lynda Hobson

BARNES & NOBLE BOOKS

A DIVISION OF HARPER & ROW, PUBLISHERS

New York, Hagerstown, San Francisco, London

This book was originally published in France under the title
Couper les cheveux soi-même © 1976 by Solar Editeur.

First BARNES & NOBLE BOOKS edition published 1977

LIBRARY OF CONGRESS CATALOG CARD NUMBER: 77–51

ISBN: 0-06-463459-0

82 83 84 85 86   10 9 8 7 6 5

Contents

Introduction
SHORT

BLUNT

LAYERED

MEN'S STYLES

Introduction

Fourteen years in the hairdressing business have taught me that every so often women love to cut a bit of hair here and there; sometimes they have to do it in an emergency. This kind of snipping away can occasionally damage the hair—making it a little uneven or really jagged—and it can often lead to total calamities.

I have seen a lot of unexpected results from these untimely and clumsy clipping sessions—and a few real catastrophes. I remember, for example, a young woman who had magnificent long hair and wanted it just a little bit shorter; after trying again and again to even it off and finding that all she had to show for her efforts was an ultrashort haircut, she ran desperately to the first hairdresser she could find to fix up the mess she had made. There is also her friend who wants her hair cut "just a little" and her child who refuses to go to the barber or hairdresser; and let's not forget her husband who is afraid of wasting too much time at the barber but really needs a few snips to at least look presentable. Finally, there is the desire that suddenly overwhelms you to give yourself a trim—to tidy your hair up a little.

All right, then, if you have to cut your own hair, do it as well as you can, try and avoid catastrophes, and, even better (why not?), manage to turn out a really good cut.

To help you achieve your goal, I put at your disposal my experience and my haircutting preferences. I have simplified the motions and operations as much as possible so that you can carry them out without difficulty and without harming your hairdo, the aim of all this being to make your hair and face as attractive as you can. Since that is the case, don't jump to the conclusion that the instruction in this book (which is by no means intended to be exhaustive) can replace the attentions of a professional hairdresser.

This book will still be useful to you even if you don't want to imitate me. It shows you how to better understand the art of hairdressing; more specifically, it teaches you how to communicate with your hairdresser—which isn't always easy.

Short Cut
with Bangs
Combed to the Side

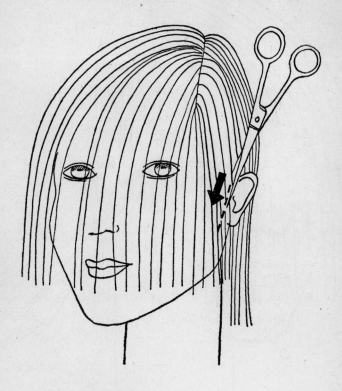

Bring the hair forward over the face starting from the crown. Then make a part on the side you want back to the crown. As shown in the illustration, cut the hair around the ear at the level of the inner edge of the ear, not the outside rim.

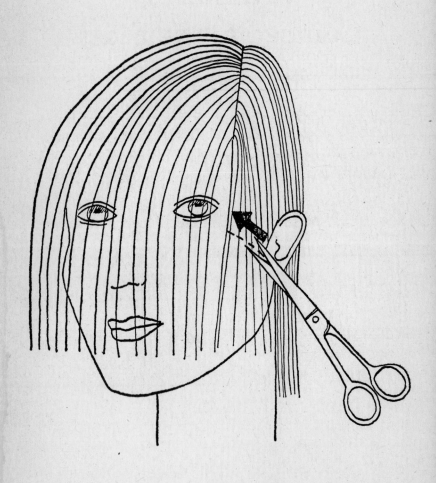

Cut along the temple, following the slanting dotted line, thus forming a triangle with the ear.

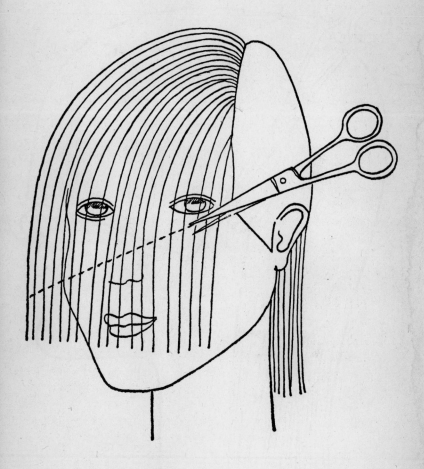

Cut the hair that has been brought forward over the
face, following the slanting dotted line, going from the
eye on the side that is parted to the cheekbone on the
opposite side of the face.

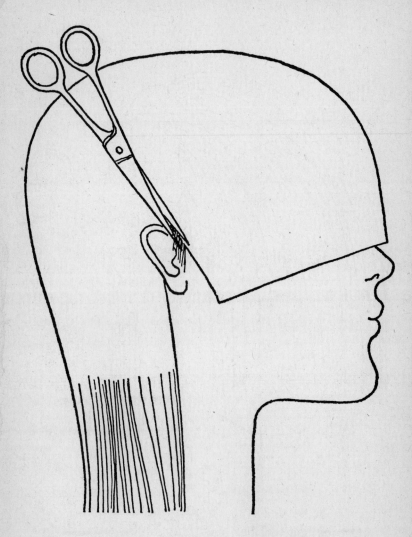

Cut the hair around the other ear, following the interior edge. This drawing clearly shows you the cut at this stage.

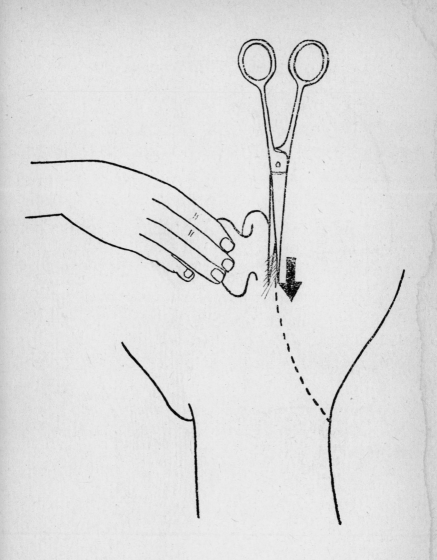

Gently bend the ear forward and even out what you
have cut so far, following the curve outlined in the
drawing.

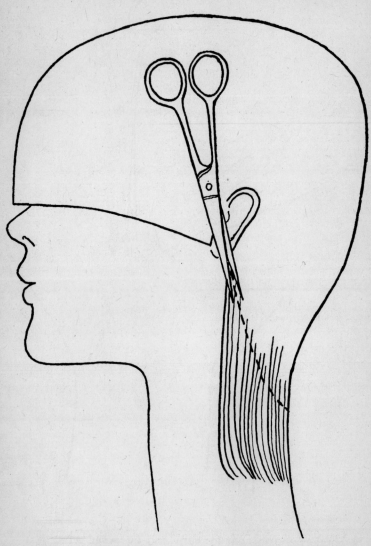

Cut along the dotted line that shows the nape of the neck.

12

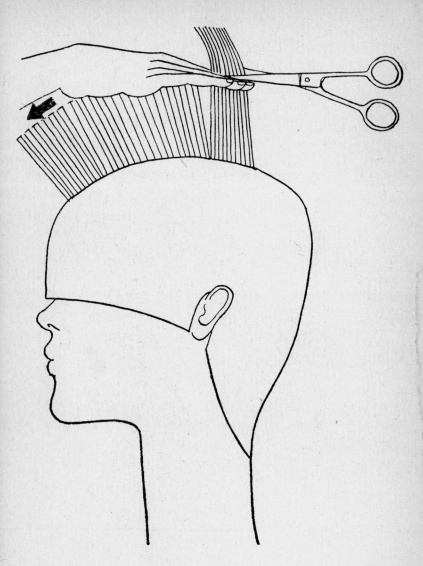

Estimate the length of the top. Section by section, cut all the hair on the top of the head the same length without changing the line you have already cut.

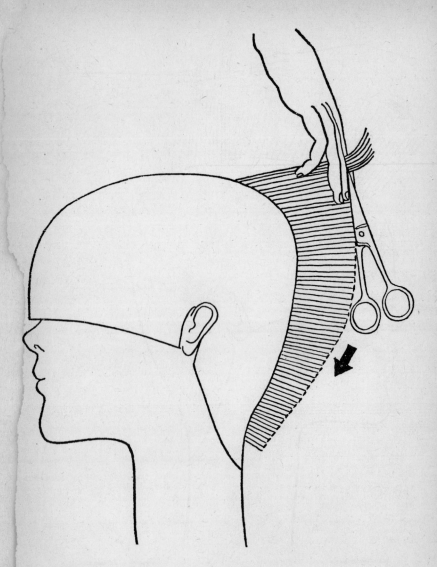

Cut the hair along the nape of the neck slightly shorter, as shown in the illustration, so that it will be thin-
ner.

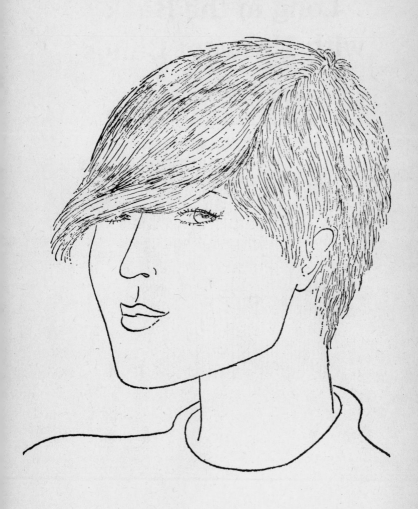

And here's the final result.

Short Cut,
Long in the Back,
with Upswept Bangs

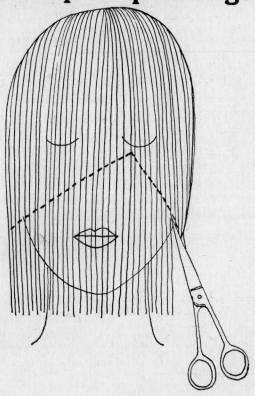

Bring the hair forward from the crown, then cut along the dotted line from one ear to the other. (This hairstyle covers the ears.)

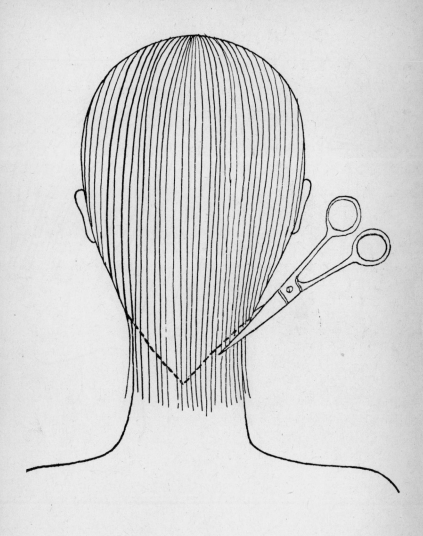

In the back, cut along the dotted line, making sure that you start low enough to cover your hairline.

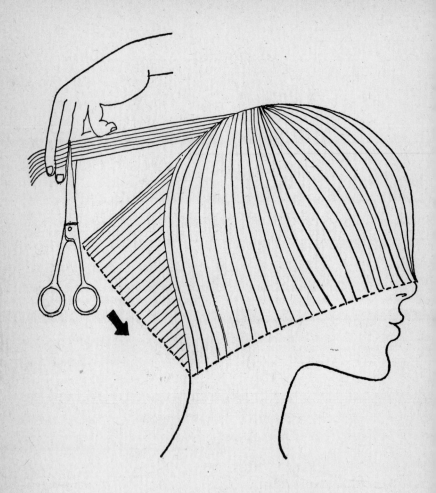

Cut the central back section, starting at the crown, the same length as the hair covering the ears; then cut it on a slant following the dotted line in the direction of the arrow.

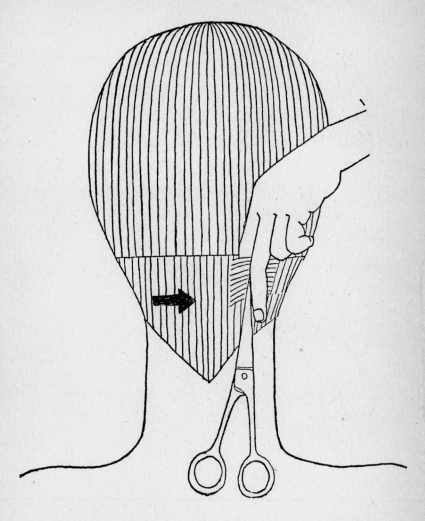

Finish cutting layers in the back, below the straight line in the drawing, going from left to right and from right to left; don't touch the central slanting cut you just finished (according to the preceding drawing).

19

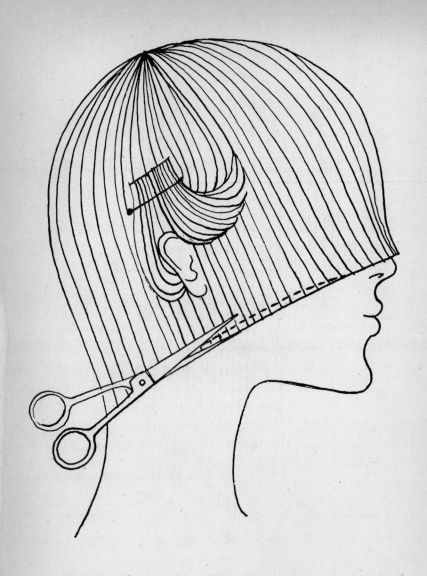

Cut the layer of hair underneath a shade shorter (¼ inch) as shown in the drawing so that the cut will look very clean.

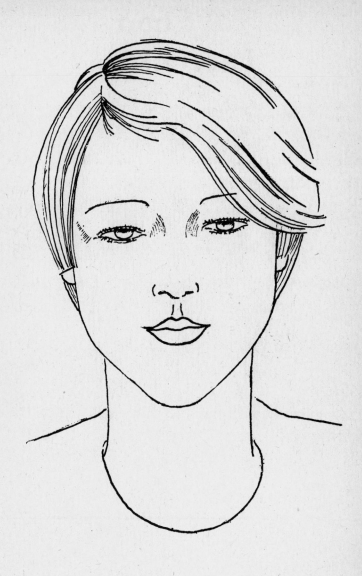

And here's the final result.

A Short
Layered Cut

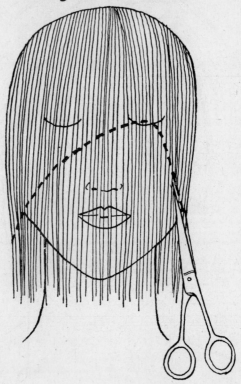

Starting from the crown, bring down over the face all
the hair from the top front of the head and cut along
the dotted line as shown in the drawing, forming a
kind of asymmetrical triangle. It is very important to
follow this line exactly in order to get the hair to flow
gently to the right (or to the left if you reverse the
direction of the cut).

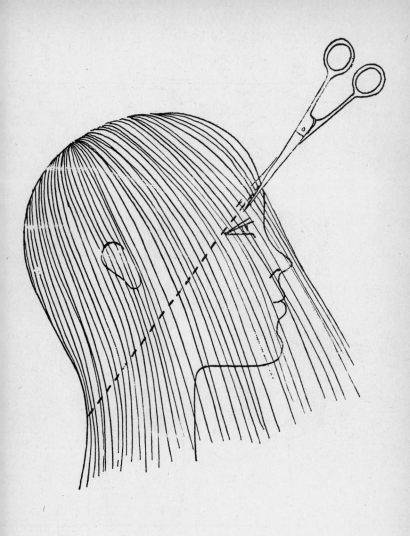

Cut along the line marked out by the dots.

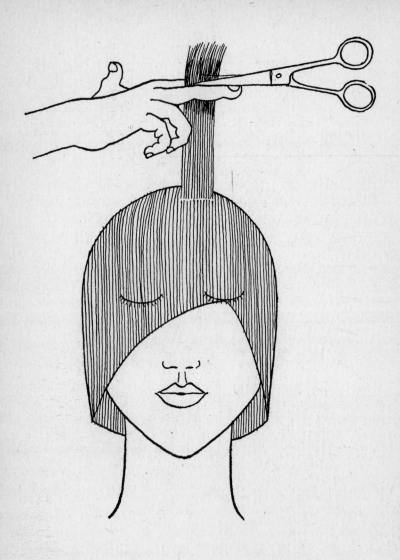

Don't recut the front layer. Cut all the hair the same length as the shortest hair of the bangs, as shown by the illustration.

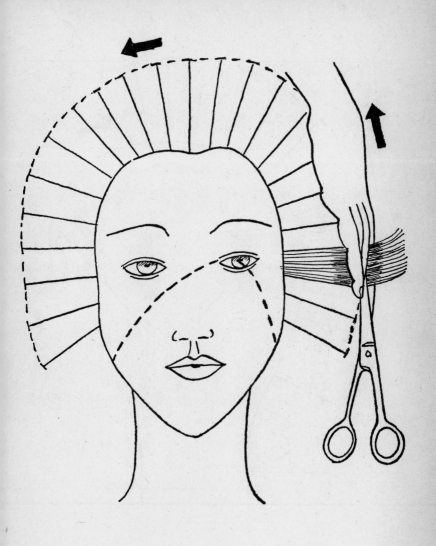

Continue cutting, holding up each lock of hair, as shown by the above drawing.

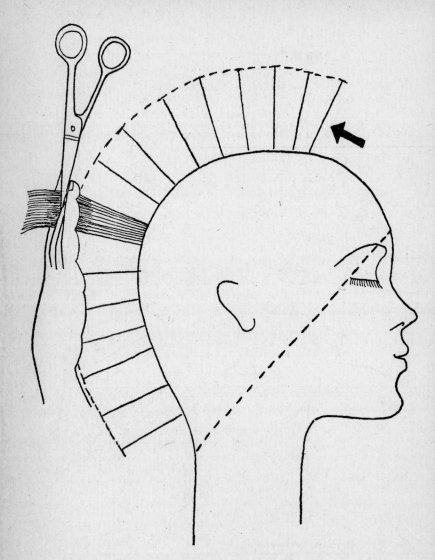

This drawing, with the head in profile, shows the way you should cut and the complete symmetry of the haircut.

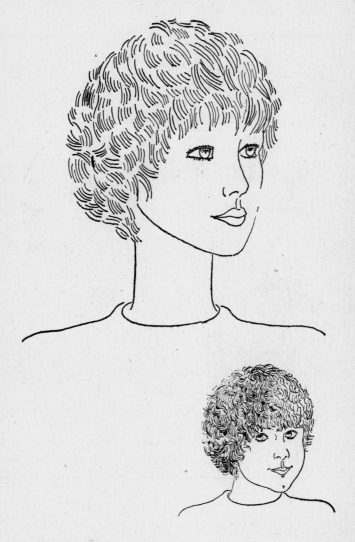

And here's the final result on curly hair combed forward.
The same hairstyle on a child.

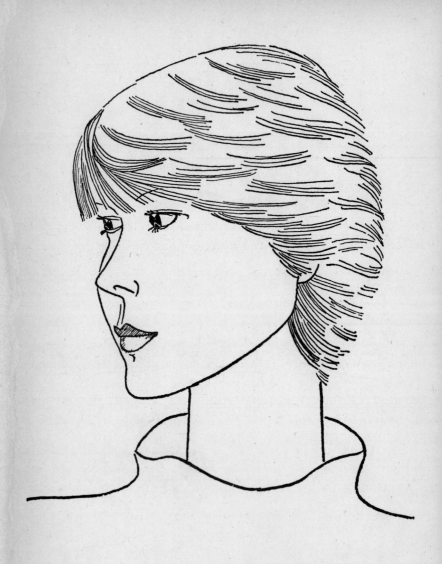

And here's the final result on straight hair lightly
brushed back.

Short Cut
à la Jean Seberg

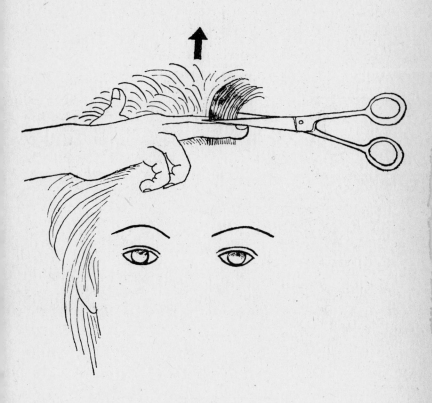

Cut the front layer the length you want—it can vary
from ¼ to 1½ inches.

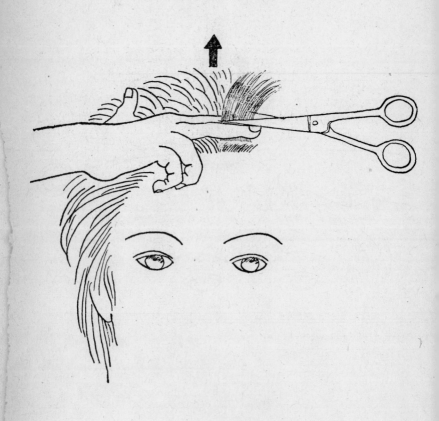

Cut the rest of the hair the same length.

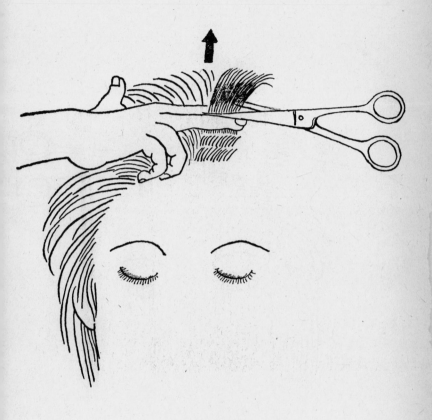

Continue cutting, always using the hair you have just cut as a guide.

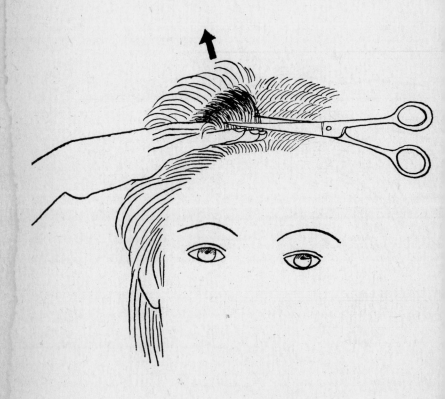

Keep cutting the hair as shown by the drawing; there shouldn't be any problems here.

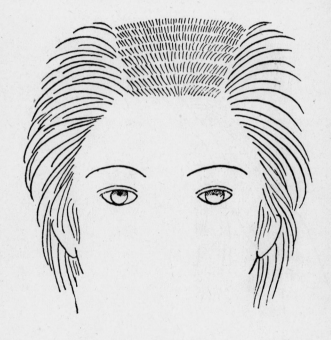

Here is a section of the finished cut.

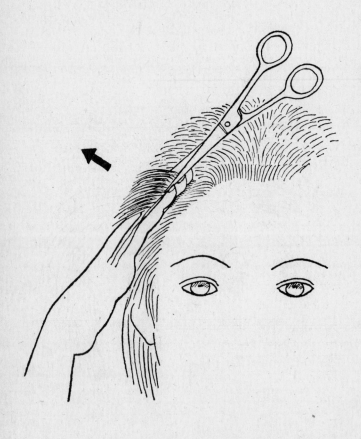

Continue cutting patiently—and be careful to keep
the length the same all over.

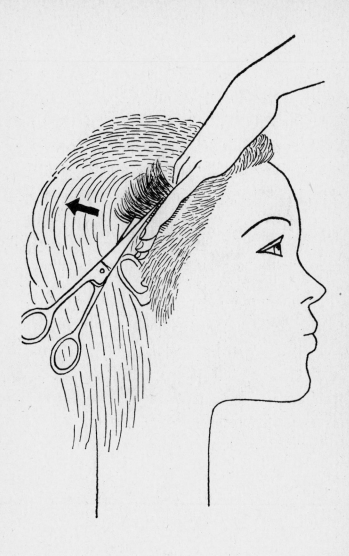

Follow the order of cutting indicated by the diagram
in order to keep the hair very even.

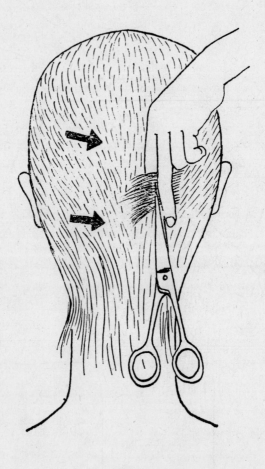

When you reach the back of the head, continue cutting, in the direction indicated by the hand, the scissors, and the arrows.

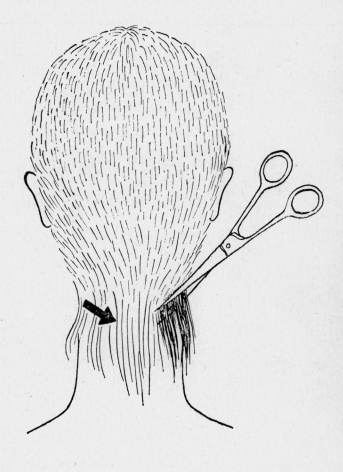

Then cut the hair on the nape of the neck the length you want it, making sure that you cover the hairline.

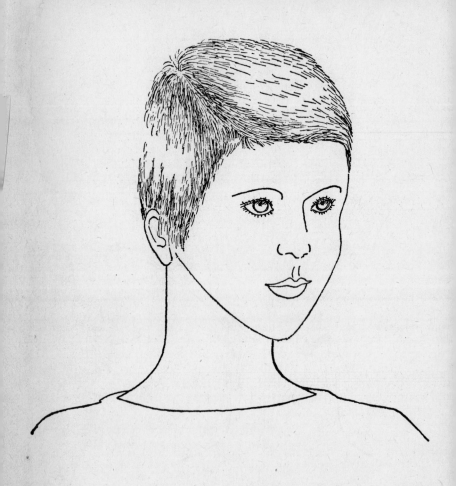

And here's the final result with the hair combed forward.

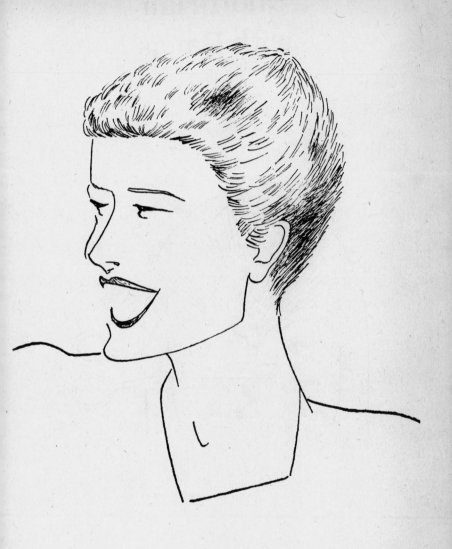

And the final result with the hair brushed back.

Short Hair
with Bangs

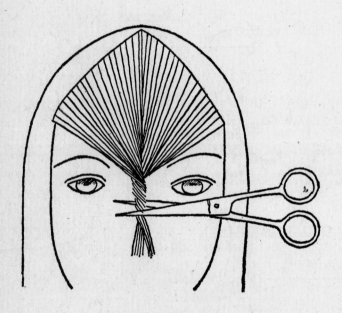

Make a part and form a triangle as indicated in the drawing. Gather the hair and twist it together; cut it cleanly at the bridge of the nose.

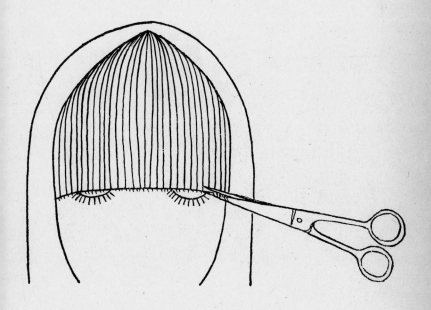

Even off the bangs out to the ears; don't destroy the
clean line by a slipup.

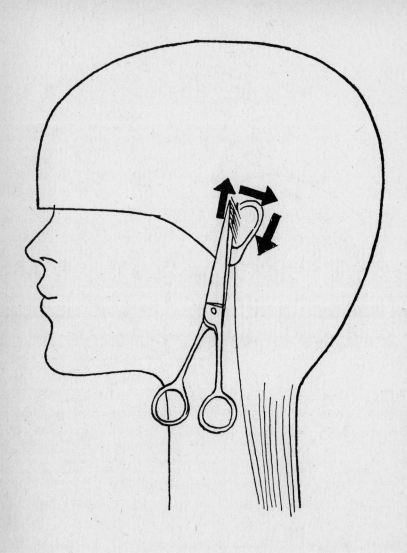

The cut goes around the ear, as shown by the arrows on the drawing.

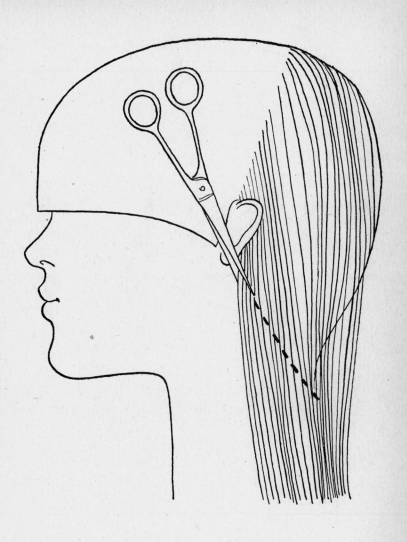

Continue cutting the sides following the dotted line.

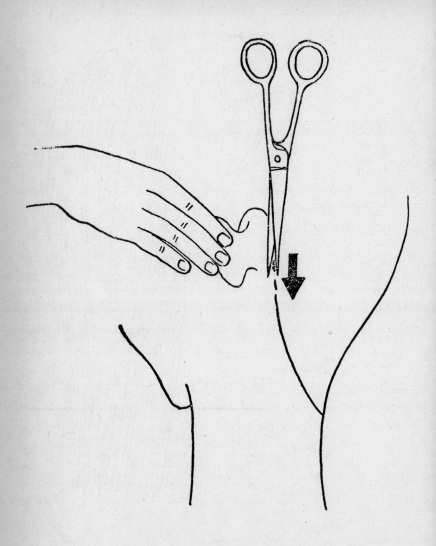

Gently bend the ear forward and even off the cut
without altering the line you have made.

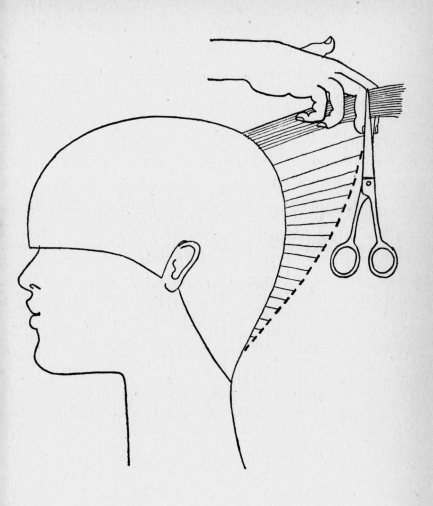

From the crown to the nape of the neck, cut the hair on the back of the head to form a gentle curve or a straight line, 2 inches long at the crown and ½ inch long at the nape of the neck.

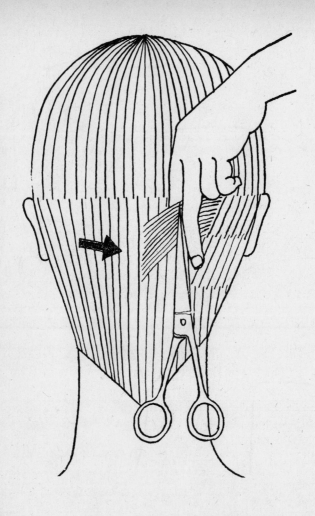

The hair around the top of the head is unchanged, and all the hair of the crown is the same length. Below this "skullcap" cut section by section starting from the ear and going toward the center, as shown by the drawing. Then start from the other ear and go toward the center as you did on the other side.

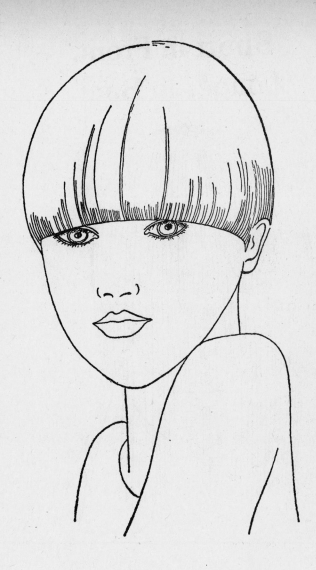

And here's the final result.

Short in Front, Longer in Back

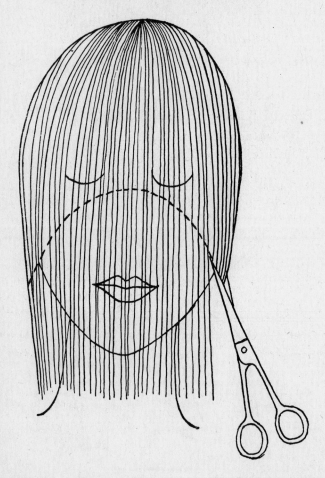

Bring the hair forward from the crown and cut along the dotted line, from one earlobe to the other, forming a curve that passes over the bridge of the nose.

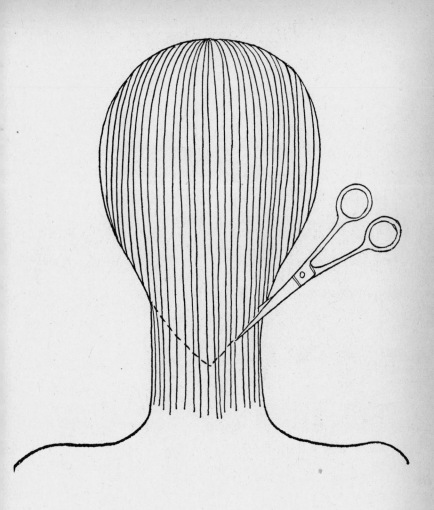

Outline the nape of the neck, keeping the hairline in mind, by following a line near or similar to the one that is shown by the dotted line.

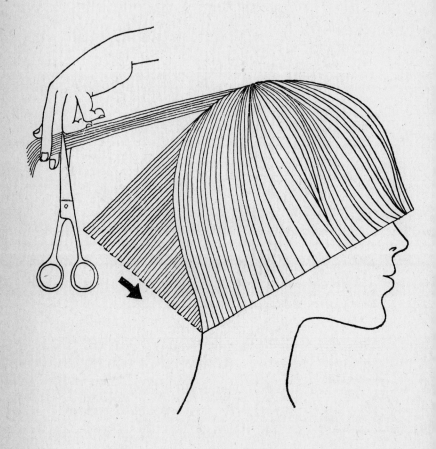

Starting from the crown, cut the hair the length of the sides at ear level. Then cut all the rest of the hair on a slant going toward the nape of the neck, as shown by the drawing.

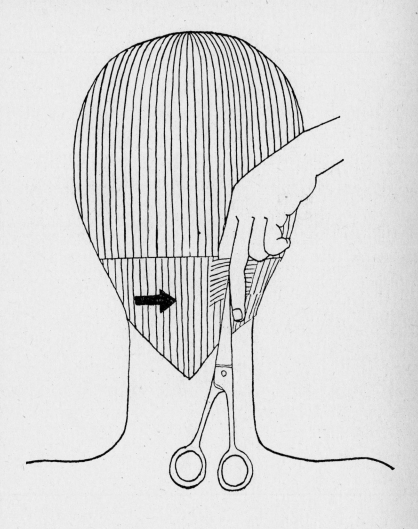

Finish cutting layers from left to right and from right to left underneath the line drawn in the illustration that shows where the hair which is all one length ends.

51

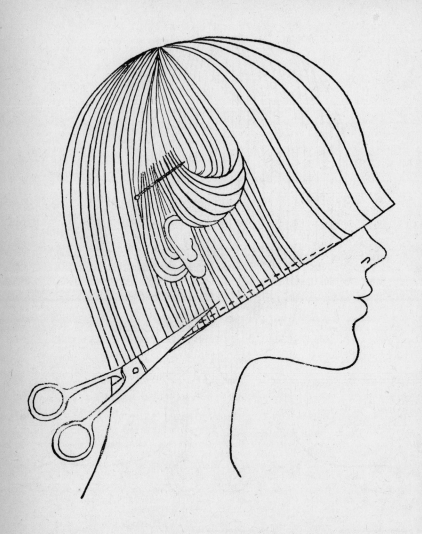

Lift up and clip the top layer of the hair in front of and behind the ear, and cut the loose hair ¼ inch shorter than the top layer so that the cut will be clean.

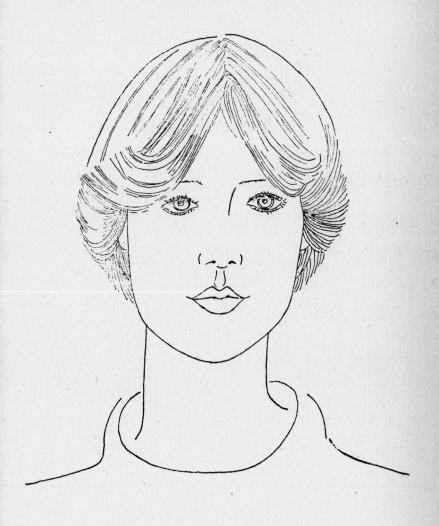

And here's the final result with the hair lightly turned up.

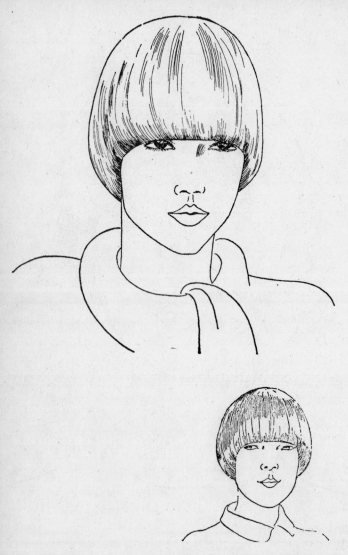

And here's the final result with the hair brought forward framing the face.
The result on a child.

Blunt Cut
with Bangs

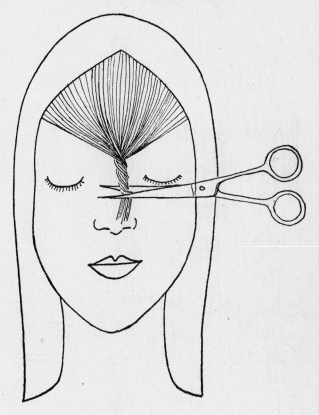

Make a part in the middle and then form a triangle, as shown by the drawing.

The farther the top of the triangle is from the forehead, the thicker the bangs.

Twist the ends of the hair together as indicated, and cut neatly at the bridge of the nose.

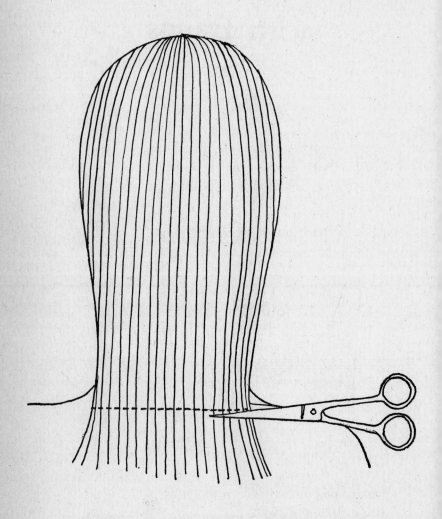

Cut the hair in the back the length you want it, along a straight line.

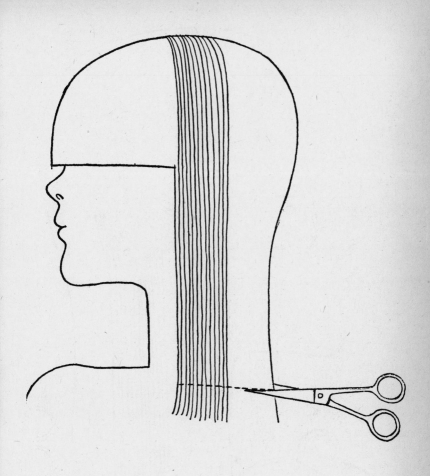

Cut the sides the same length as the back, along a straight line.

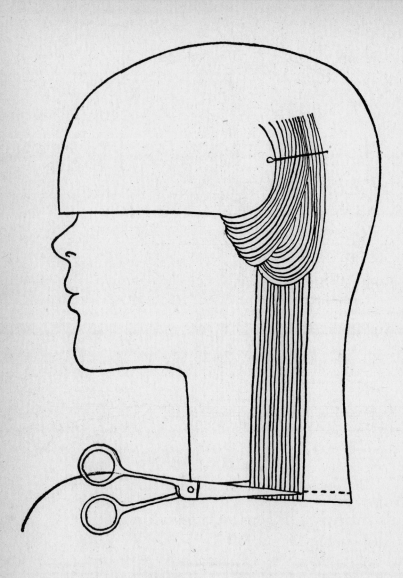

To make the cut neat, lift up and clip the sides, and then cut the hair that is loose ¼ inch shorter than the rest.

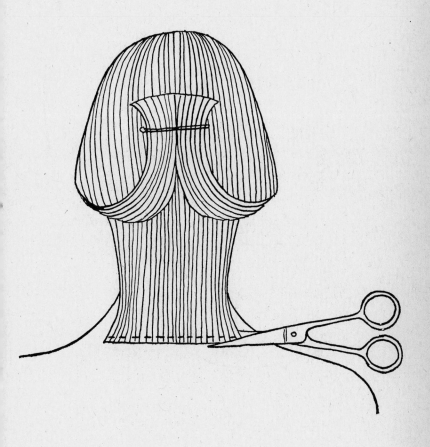

Lift up and clip the top layer of hair and cut the layer underneath ¼ inch shorter than the top layer.

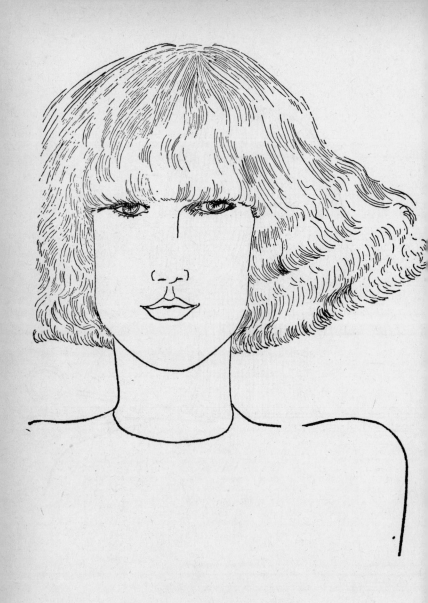

And here's the final result with curly hair.

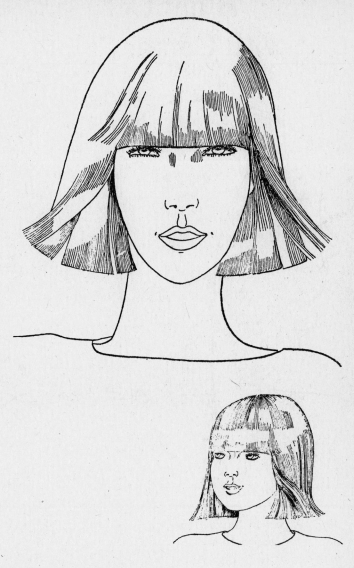

And with straight hair.
And here's the way it looks on a little girl.

Blunt Cut
with Center Part

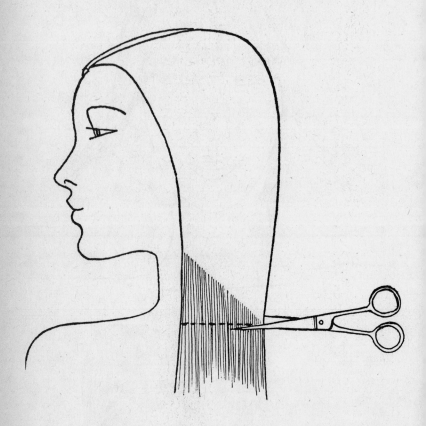

Make a part in the middle back to the crown. Bring the hair from both sides of the face forward; then, with the head turned sideways and the shoulders facing front, cut the hair straight across the length you want it.

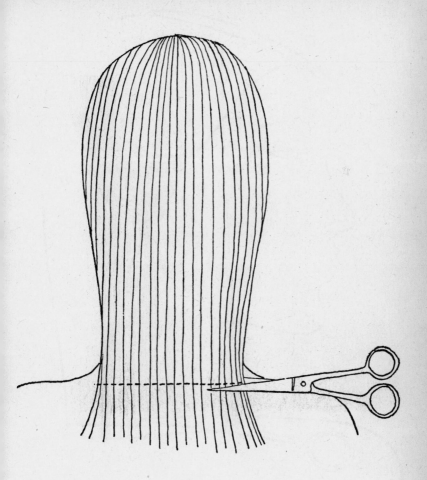

Cut the hair in the back absolutely straight across the same length as the sides.

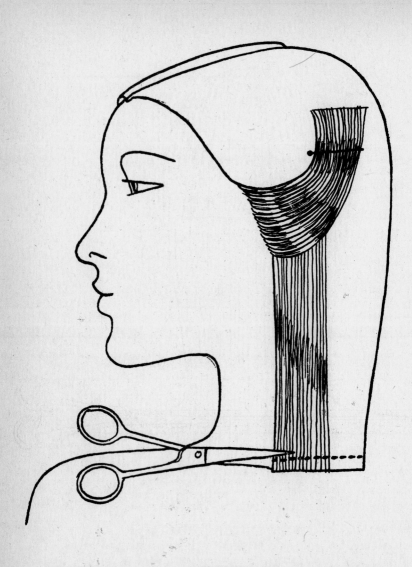

To make the line of the cut very clean, lift up and clip the hair from the forehead at the sides, as shown in the drawing, and cut the loose hair ¼ inch shorter than the hair you have clipped up.

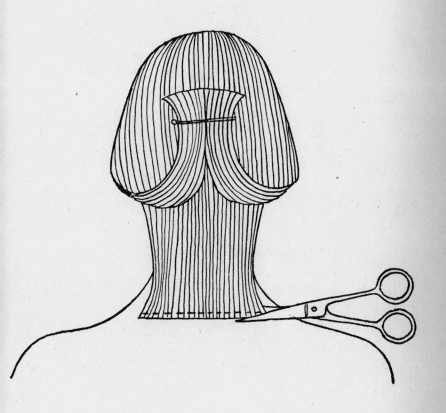

In the back, lift up and clip the top layer of hair, and
cut the loose hair ¼ inch shorter, as you just did with
the sides.

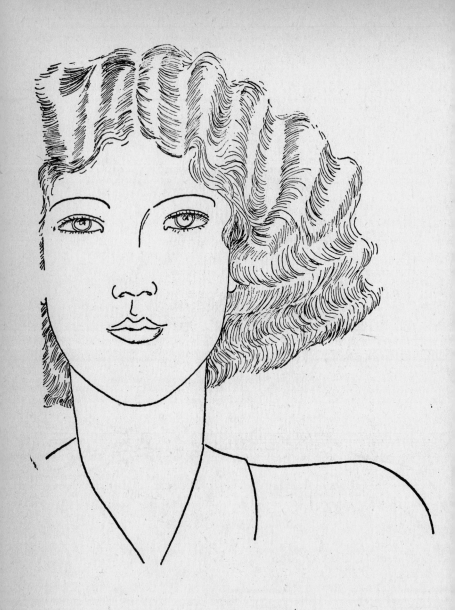

And here's the final result on curly hair.

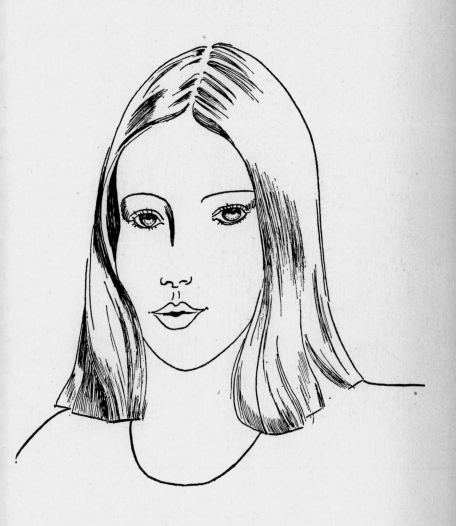

And on straight hair.

Blunt Cut
with Side Part

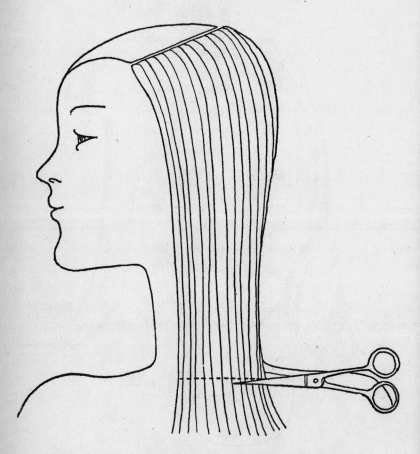

Make a part on the side the way you want it; then, with your head turned sideways and your shoulders facing front, cut the side with the part along the straight dotted line.

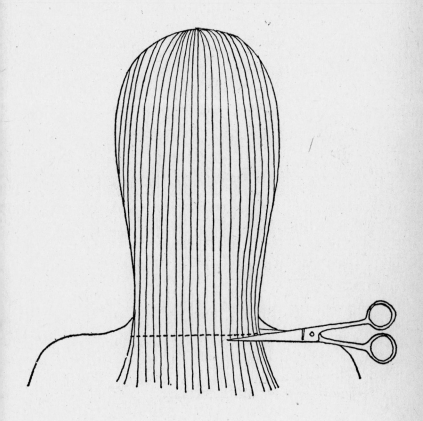

In the back, cut straight across the same length as the
sides, as shown in the drawing.

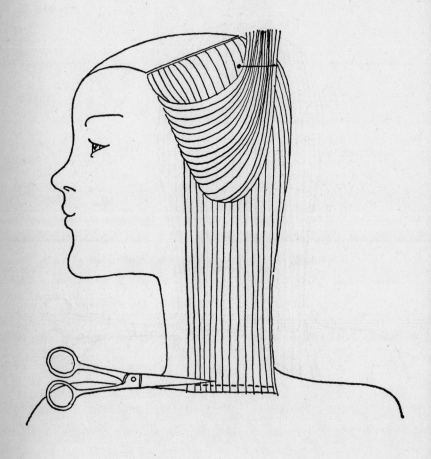

To make the cut clean, lift up and clip the top layers
and trim the loose hair ¼ inch.

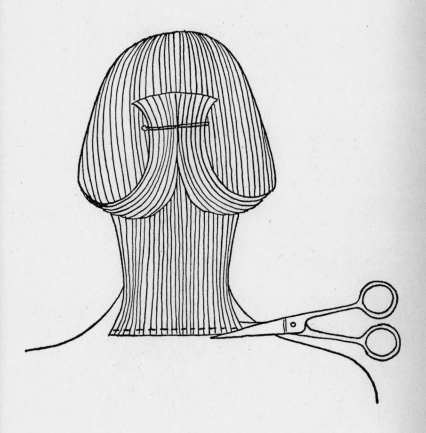

The illustration is clean trim the loose hair ¼ inch.

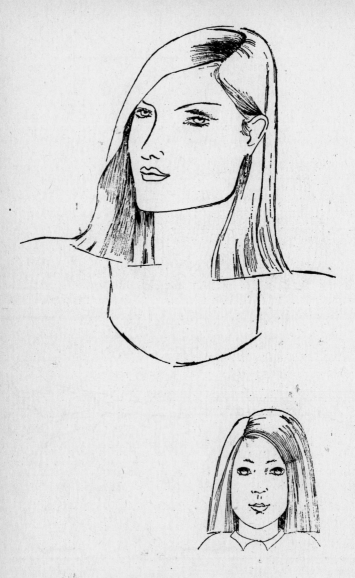

And here's the final result on straight hair.
Here's how it looks on a little girl.

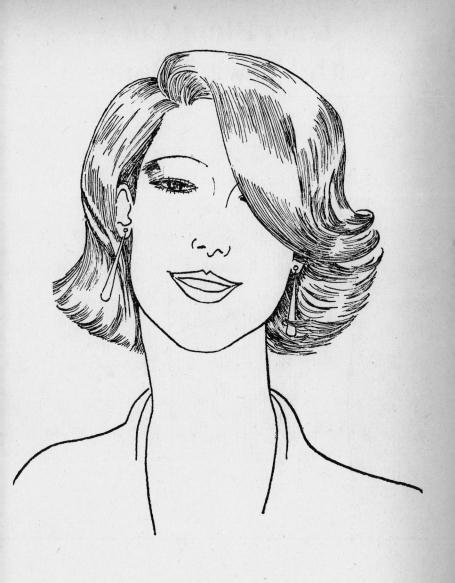

And on fluffy hair gently turned up.

Long Blunt Cut
with Upswept Bangs

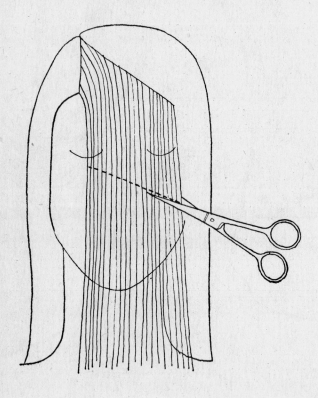

Make a part on the side. Bring the hair forward. Form
a triangle as shown in the drawing; then cut following
the slanting dotted line in the direction recommended
—from bottom to top.

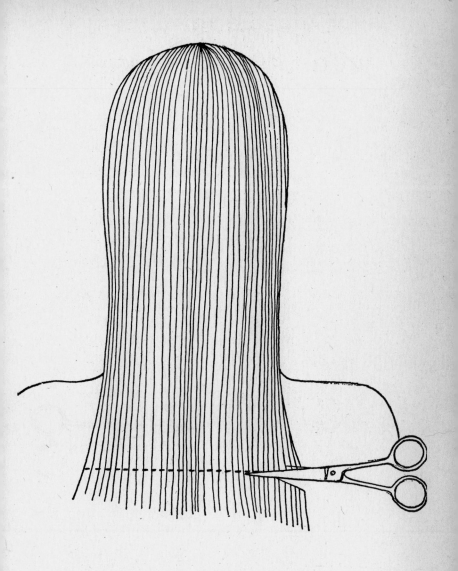

Cut the hair in the back the length you want it, along a straight line.

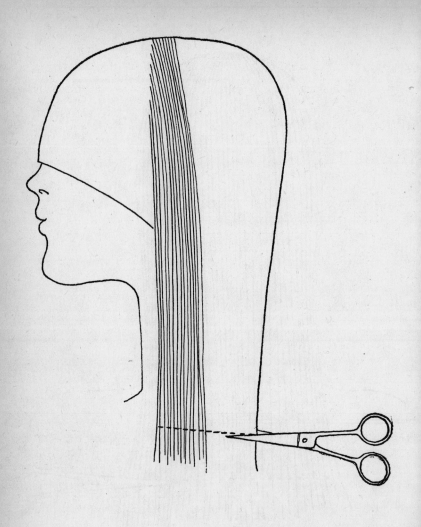

Continue cutting straight across on the sides.

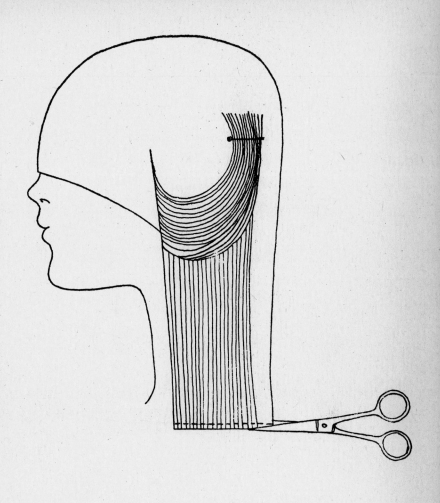

Lift up and clip the top layer of hair, as shown in the
drawing, and trim the bottom layer ¼ inch.

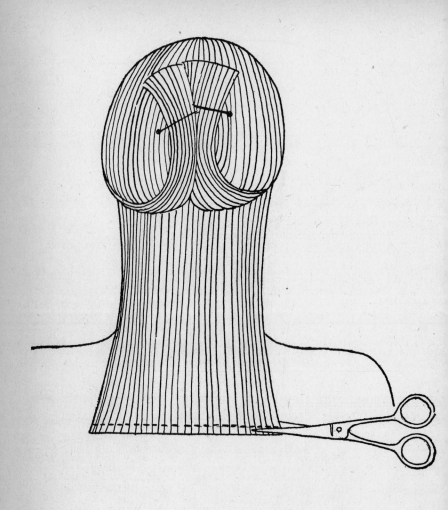

Do the same thing in the back so that the cut will be clean.

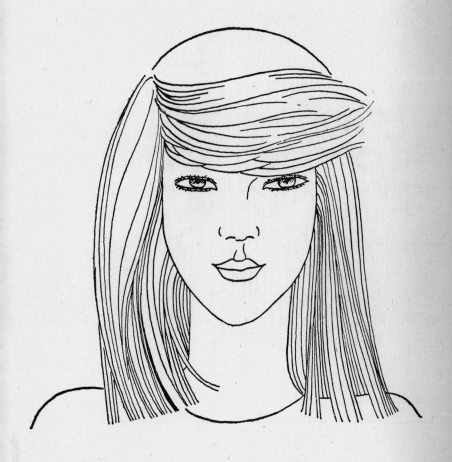

And here's the final result of this long blunt cut with
swept-up bangs.

The Stone Cut

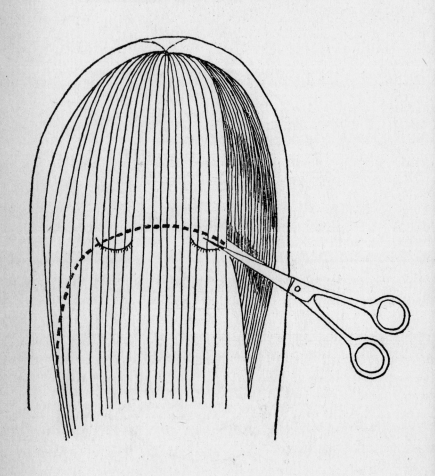

Bring the hair from the crown down over the face. Then cut following the arc of the circle traced by the dotted line, below the eyebrows.

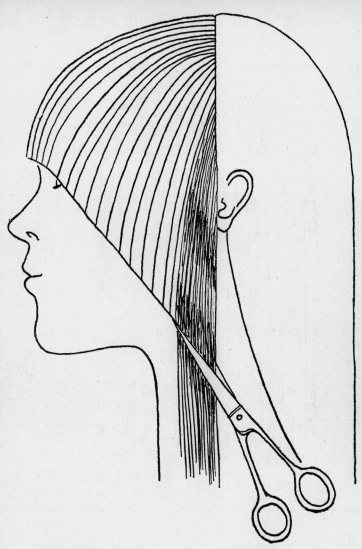

With the head turned sideways and the shoulders facing front, continue the slanting line of the front along
the sides, as shown by the drawing.

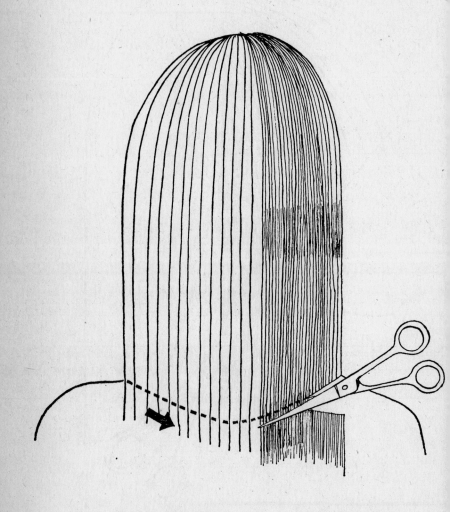

In the back, cut along the gentle curve that has been outlined, starting from one side and then from the other, as shown by the scissors and the arrow.

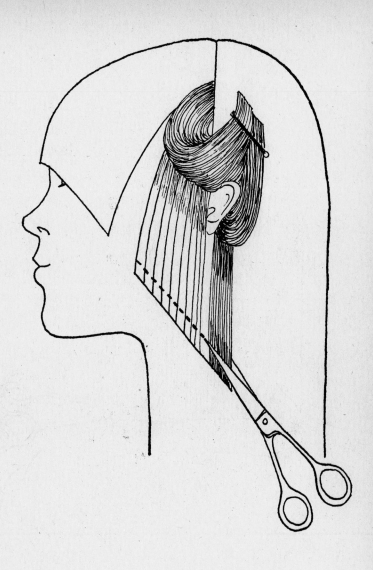

Then, to make the cut clean, lift up and clip the top
layer of hair, and trim the bottom layer ¼ inch.

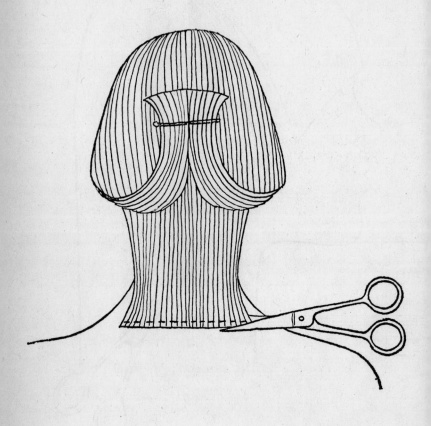

Do the same in the back.

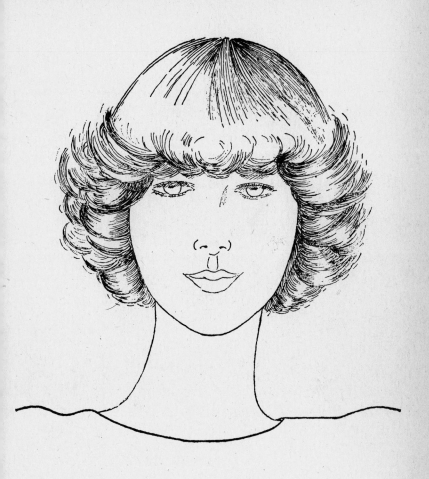

And here's the result on wavy hair lightly turned up.

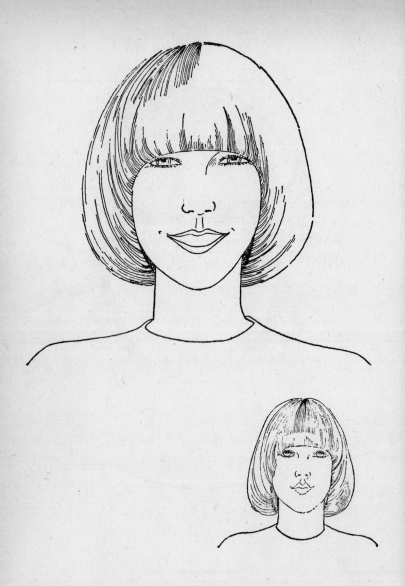

And on straight hair with the hair brought forward
gently framing the face.
The same hairdo on a child.

Long Layered Cut
à la Jane Fonda

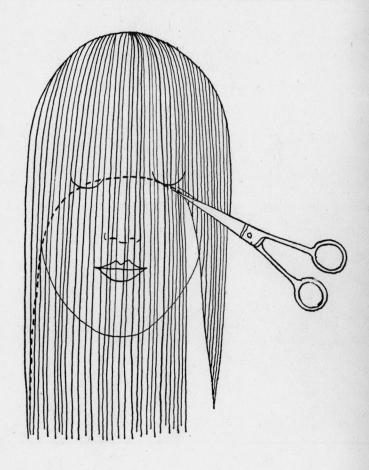

Bring the hair from the crown down over the face and outline a curve, cutting along the dotted line.

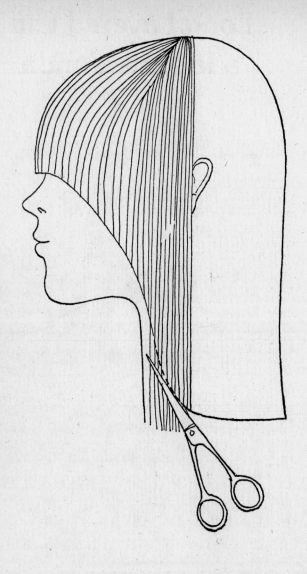

Cut the sides following the curve shown by the dotted line.

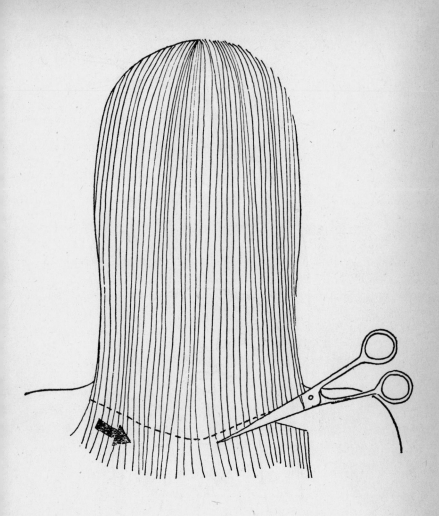

In the back, continue cutting from left to right and from right to left, as indicated by the arrow and the scissors.

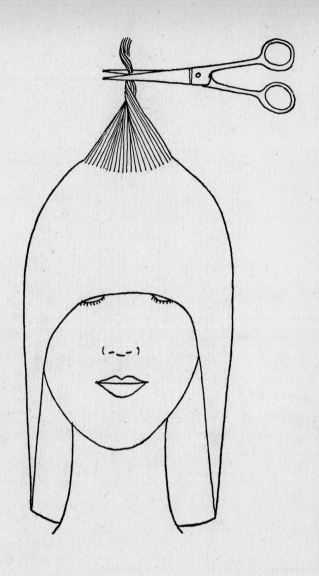

Lift up and twist together the hair of the crown; then cut it neatly so that it will be 3 to 4 inches long.

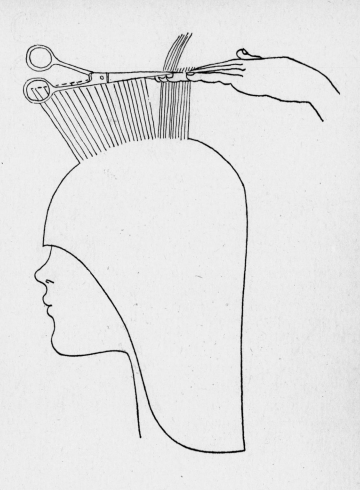

As shown in the drawing, continue the cut of the crown up to the forehead, using the central section you have just cut as a guide to the length and so on, holding each section on a slant (cut on a diagonal in the direction shown by the drawing). Don't cut the bangs again.

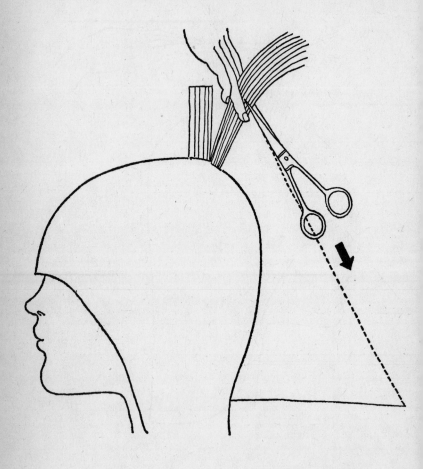

Continue cutting in the back, as shown in the drawing. The straight line of the base of the triangle repre-
sents the hair of the nape of the neck that has already
been cut held out horizontally, the better to show you
the sloping line of the cut—which forms a triangle
with this horizontal line.

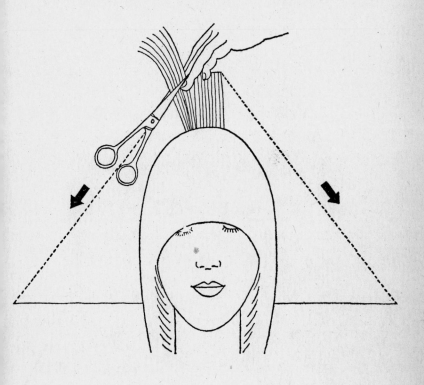

Cut the hair on the sides on the diagonal following the dotted line and the direction of the arrow starting from the crown. The horizontal line of the base shows the sides held out straight, so that the slanting line of the cut is more emphasized.

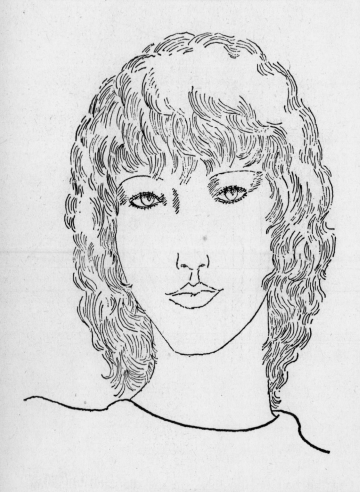

And here is the result of the Jane Fonda cut on curly
hair.

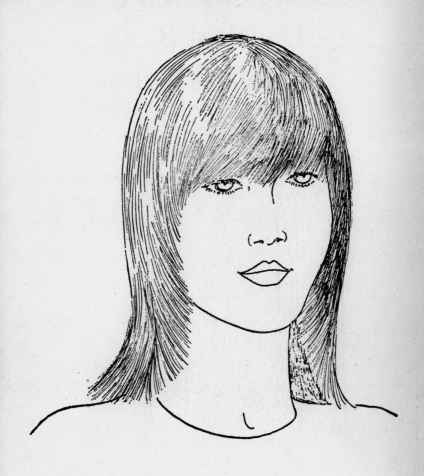

And on straight hair.

Long Layered Cut, Upswept Bangs Framing the Face

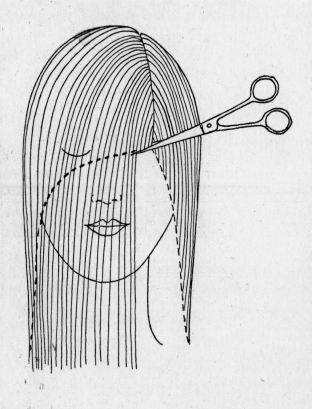

Make a part on the side you want, as shown by the drawing. Bring the hair forward over the face, then cut following the dotted line.

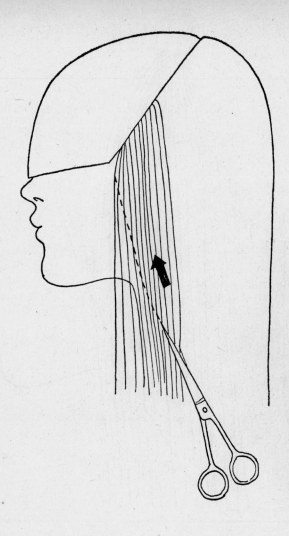

With the head facing sideways and the shoulders facing forward, the better to see the profile, cut following
the gentle curve of the dotted line.

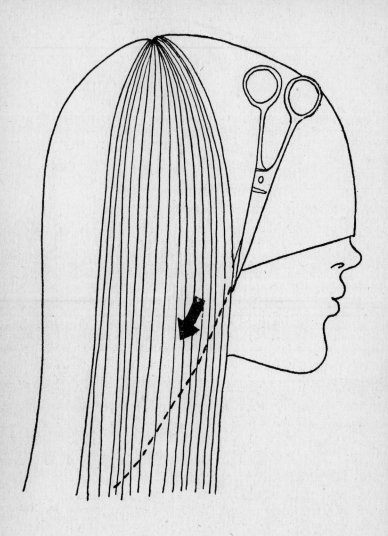

Cut the hair on the other side following the dotted
line in the direction shown by the arrow.

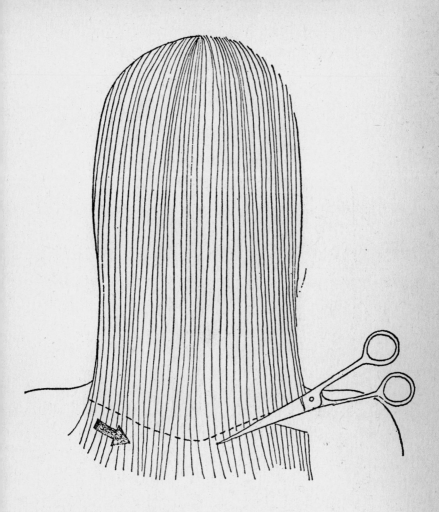

Cut the back section along the curve shown by the dotted line, from left to right and from right to left as shown by the arrow and the scissors.

Then, as recommended for some of the preceding haircuts, trim the bottom layer ¼ inch so that the cut will be clean.

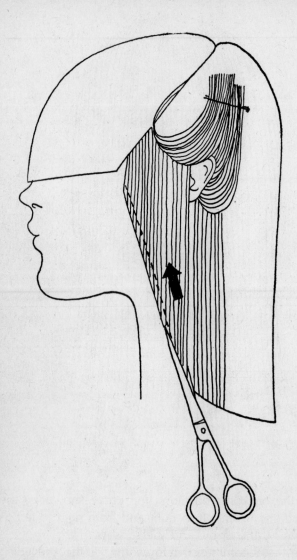

Slightly shorten the bottom layer after you have lifted up and pinned the top layer. Cut from bottom to top in the direction of the arrow.

100

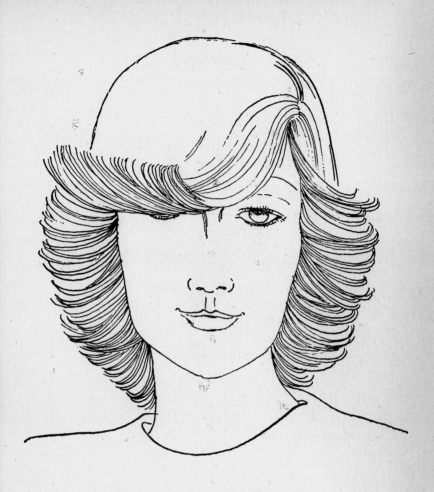

And there's the final result with the hair turned up. This coiffure can also be very attractive with the hair turned under.

Medium-Length
Layered Cut

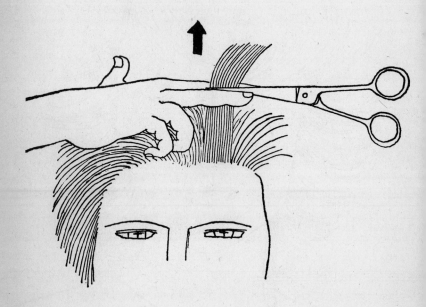

Cut the top section about 2½ to 3 inches long from front to back.

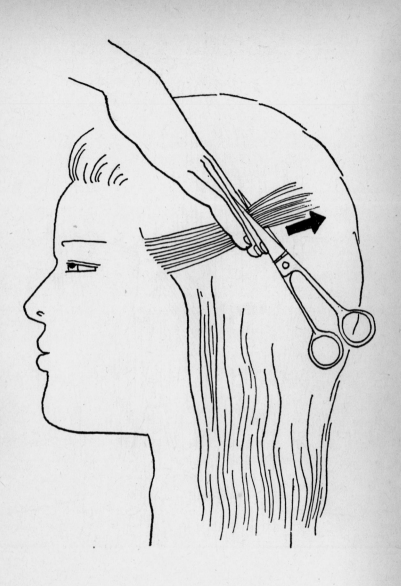

Cut the sides the same length in the direction of the
arrow.

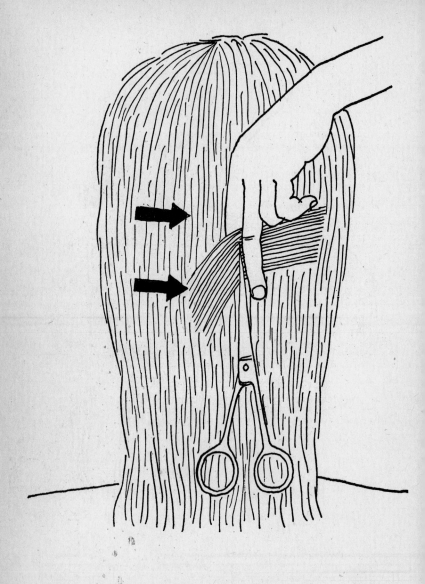

In the back, go from left to right and right to left, cutting section by section the same length.

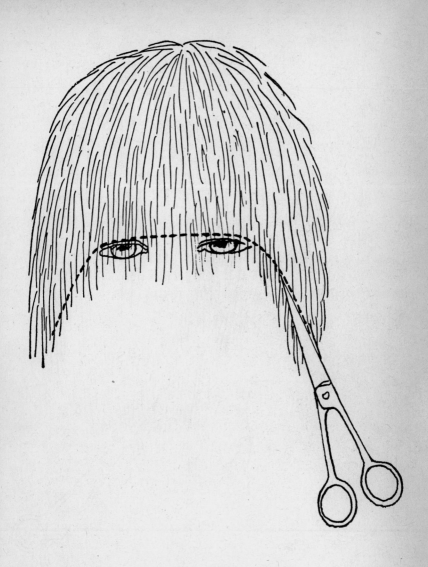

Bring all the hair forward starting from the crown;
then cut along the dotted line.

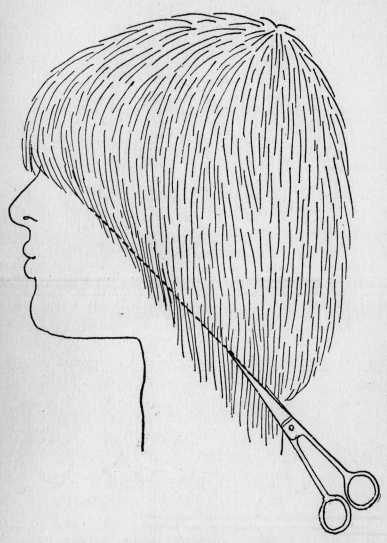

Even off the sides from left to right following the dotted line from bottom to top.

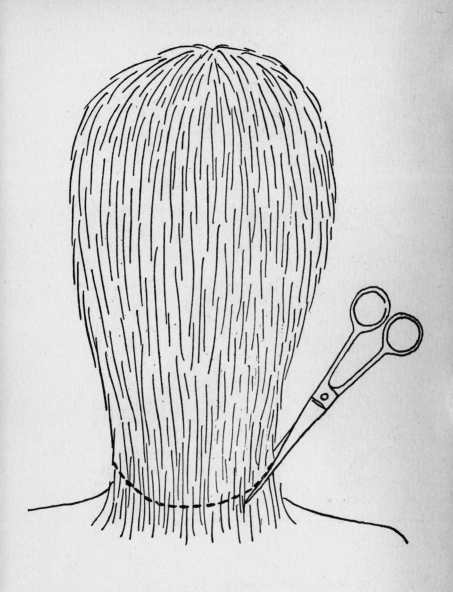

Even off the nape of the neck.

107

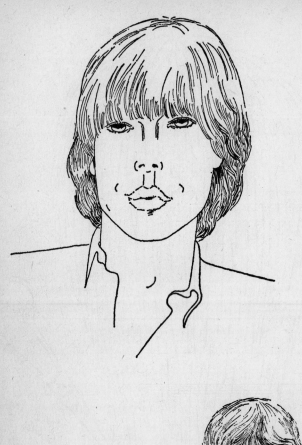

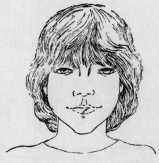

And here's the final result.
The same cut on a little boy.

Ivy League Look

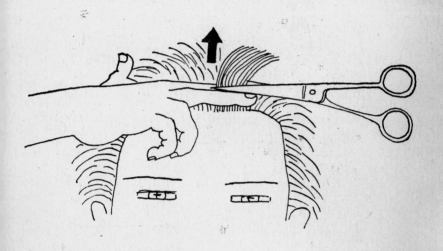

Cut the hair at the forehead ¾ to 1¼ inches long—
it's up to you. Then use the hair that you've cut as a
guide to length in cutting the rest of the hair. Cut in
the direction shown by the arrow.

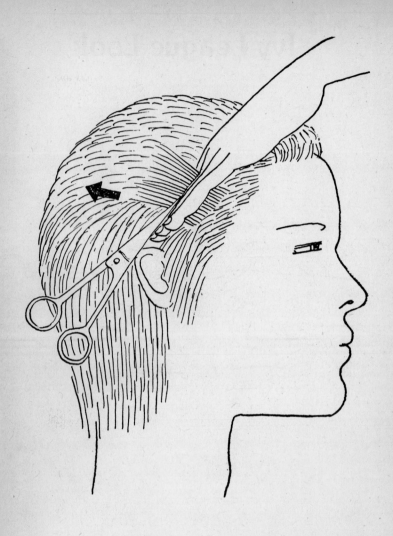

On the sides cut the hair the same length, section by
section, in the direction of the arrow.

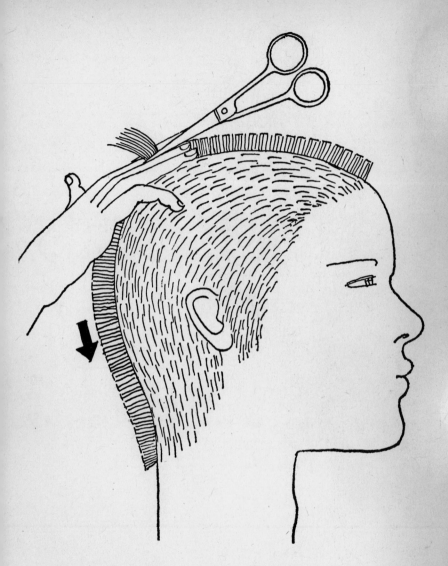

The hair standing up in this drawing shows that the cut is the same length all over (when it is cut section by section).

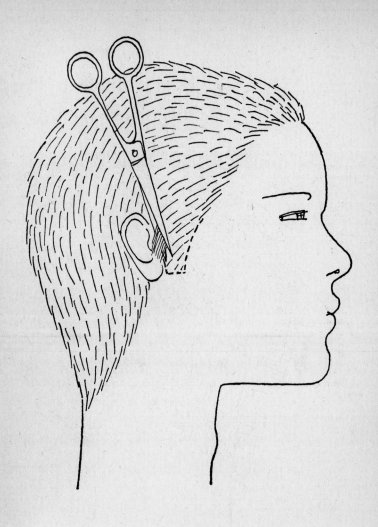

Cut, outlining the curve of the ear as shown in the drawing.

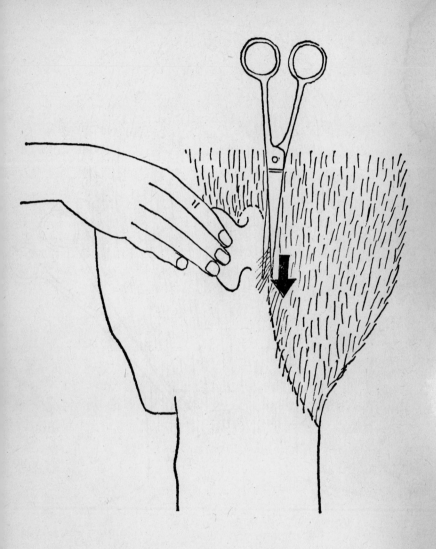

Even off the hair behind the ear as shown by the scissors and arrow.

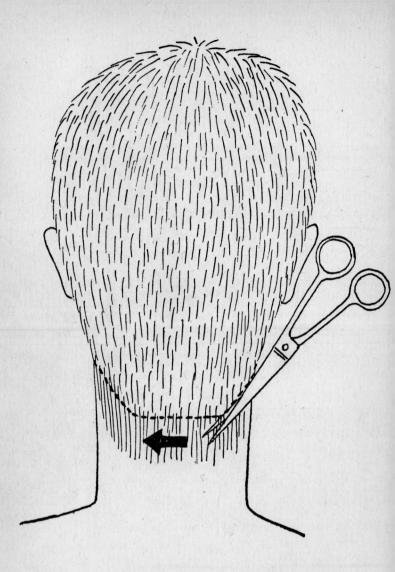

Cut the hair of the nape of the neck along the line
shown by the drawing, following a line you want, or
along a line determined by the hairline.

114

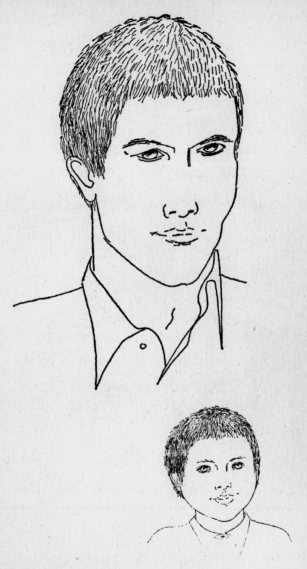

And here's the final result.
The Ivy League cut on a little boy.

Layered Cut
with Side Part

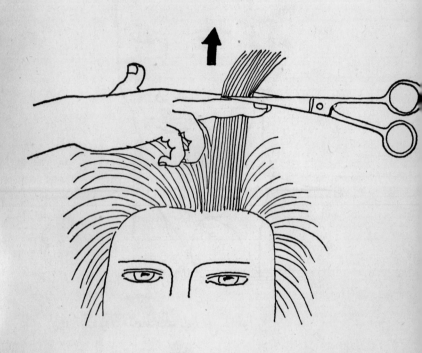

Cut the hair 1½ to 2 inches long (it's up to you), beginning with the hair at the forehead and working back to the crown and so on all around the head.

116

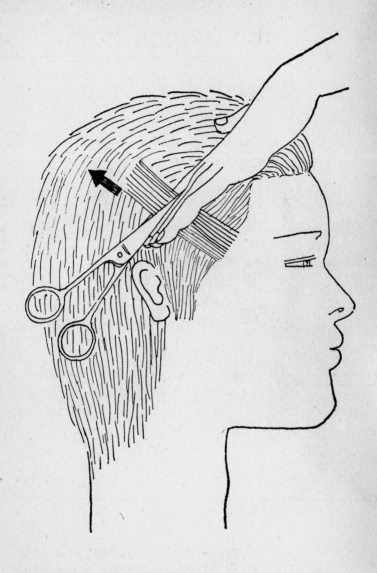

Cut the sides the same length, following the arrow.

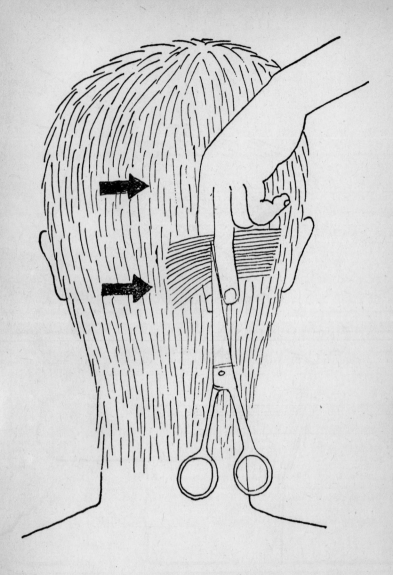

In the back, always cut section by section the same length, from left to right and from right to left in the direction of the arrow.

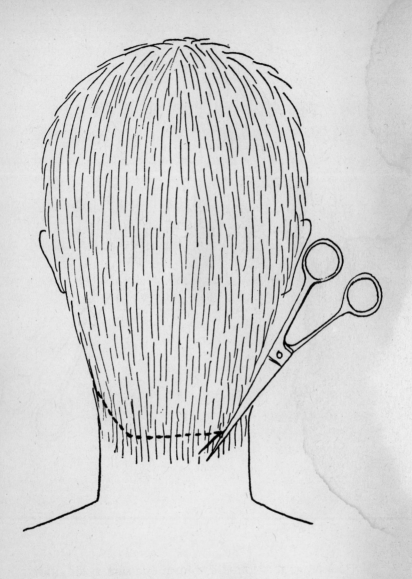

Even off the nape of the neck.

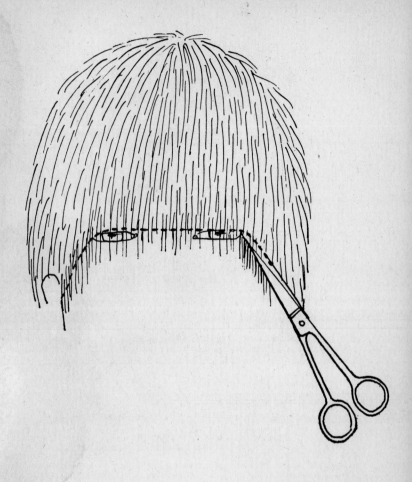

Cut along the dotted line from one side to the other;
then even it off at midear level, as shown by the final
result.

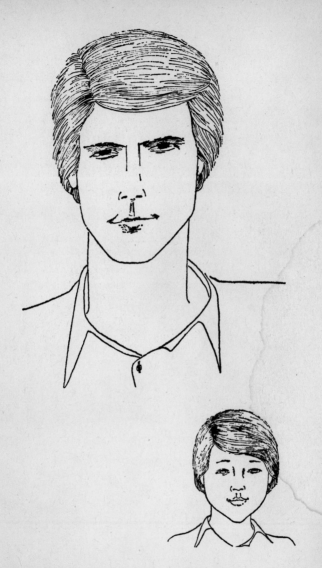

Make a part on the side you want—and here's the
final result.
The same style on a little boy.

A Few
Tricks of the Trade

Use haircutting shears and avoid razors.

Cut the hair when it's wet and make any necessary adjustments when it's dry.

You should realize that a coiffure always looks better a few days after it's cut because you've got to give the hair time to fall into place.

Don't get too carried away while you're cutting! Remember that you can always make your hair shorter but it's impossible to make it longer again.
If you want to give yourself bangs, make a part in the middle; then make a triangle—high or low, large or small, according to the width and thickness of the bangs you want. (If you have a broad face, make the triangle narrow; if you have a thin face, make the triangle wide.)

Take the hair that you have separated for the bangs and twist it together in the middle. Then cut it neatly ½ inch below the bridge of the nose. (See illustration for blunt cut with bangs, page 55.)

To trim bangs you already have, stand in front of your mirror, wet and comb down the bangs. Don't twist the hair. Shorten the bangs slightly following the initial outline, and don't forget that dry hair looks shorter than wet hair.

To cut the sides of a medium-length hairstyle, turn the head sideways while the shoulders face forward, so that you won't be hindered by the shoulders and also so that you can cut the hair on a slant. If you cut your hair yourself, you can use two mirrors or choose the position in which you feel most comfortable.

To make sure that the cut is symmetrical, put your hands up to your temples and smooth down both sides at once. Even if there is only a slight difference in length, you will easily notice it, and that will help you avoid those successive evenings off that can lead to short hair without your realizing it.

To have swept-up bangs, make a part on the side and form a triangle—higher or lower according to how thick you want the bangs—(see the illustrations for blunt cut with swept-up bangs, page 74). Bring the hair of this triangle forward and put the rest of the hair behind the ears.

Then cut on a slant, starting from the part, from eye level over to the opposite cheek.

If you want to recut the nape of the neck and you have short hair, wet the hair and smooth it down; then, with the help of two mirrors, cut the hair the length you want without changing the original outline.

If you have medium-length hair, it's better to cut it while standing so that you can more easily assess whether the length you want is the right one for your appearance (your shoulders, height, neck, and so on).